FIBROMYALGIA: FIGHTING BACK

Bev Spencer
Foreword by Glenn A. McCain, M.D.

A handbook that encourages people with fibromyalgia to fight the effects of the illness, and tells them how to do it.

Produced by LRH Publications
Printed in Canada

Copyright © 1992 by Bev Spencer

Copies of this booklet may be obtained from various fibromyalgia associations and support groups. They may also be ordered from:
LRH Publications
Box 8, Station Q
Toronto, ON M4T 2L7
Canada

Single copies $6.95, two copies $12.95. Package of two booklets *Fibromyalgia: Fighting Back* and *Coping with Fibromyalgia* $12.95. Prices for bulk orders on request. All prices include postage and taxes where applicable. For orders outside Canada, cheques or money orders should be in U.S. funds.

ISBN 0-9695785-2-0

Foreword v
Acknowledgments viii
A Personal Experience 1

1. After the Diagnosis 3
   I've Got What? 3
   At Least It's Real 3
   Still A Mystery 4
   The Good, the Bad, and the Better News 5

2. Taking Charge 6
   Know Your Enemy 6
   A Good Listener 7
   Why Me? 7
   Talking to Your Doctor 8
   Gaining Perspective 9

3. A Many-Sided Approach 9
   Why Exercise? 10
   Living With Less Pain 11
   Hurt Without Harm 12
   Pain and the Brain 13
   Fatigue and FMS 14
   Sleeping Better 14

4. Going Into Action 15
   About Exercise 15
   Listen to your Body! 18
   Getting Comfortable 19
   A Cheering Section 21

    Massage 22
    Reducing Stress 22
    Planning Your Daily Life 23
    Manage Your Memory 25
    Learning to Let Go 27

5. Assessing Your Life 29
    Your Self-Esteem 30
    You and Your Job 30
    What Are Your Options? 31
    Pardon Me, But You're Stepping on my Dreams ... 32
    Adjusting Your Expectations 32

6. From Victim to Victor 34
    Taking Stock 34
    Remember to Have Fun 35
    Laughter Is Powerful Medicine 35
    Some Diet Tips 35
    The "How Are You?" Trap 36
    Learning to Say No 37
    FMS and Intimacy 38
    Other People Hurt Too 38
    Surviving the Ups and Downs 39
    You Can Fight Fibromyalgia 39

FOREWORD

Recent years have seen great advances in our understanding of chronic pain syndromes. These advances have been led by the development of techniques which more accurately measure and hence reflect the essential human experience of pain, both in the laboratory and in the clinic.

The development of better ways to measure pain has taught investigators that the experience of chronic pain is a complex phenomenon. We learn about pain through our experience of *acute pain*. While the lessons that acute pain teach us are not entirely analogous to *chronic pain*, it is now quite clear to all of us that the perception of one's own pain is a very personal experience.

That is, pain may be felt and perceived quite differently by different individuals or by the same individual at different stages of life. No one can say that the pain of a broken leg, for example, is exactly the same for him or her as it is for someone else. Similarly, the perception of the pain from a visit to the dentist may be experienced differently by the same person in childhood and as an adult, or by a diabetic and a healthy person.

Indeed, the setting in which pain is experienced and what that pain means to the individual is of paramount importance to how severe the painful experience may be and how significantly the individual's life may be affected by it.

In medical terms, this means that those of us who seek to alleviate pain must be aware of the complexity of the painful experience. This approach has resulted in the idea that chronic pain may be viewed as consisting of a number of components which act at different levels and contribute to the final experience of what each of us perceives as pain. These dimensions of pain are sensory, affective, cognitive and behavioral in nature. Let me enlarge briefly on each of these aspects.

o *Sensory*. This indicates that the human body has a set of anatomical structures that perceive pain for us. These structures are much the same in all of us and consist of nerve endings, spinal cord reflexes and the parts of the brain that tell us about pain sensation. They include neurotransmitters and other chemical pain messengers. The sensory component of the pain experience is most easily influenced with analgesic drugs and pain killers.

- *Affective*. This indicates that beyond the pure unpleasantness of pain there is also a feeling or mood that is evoked by pain. This mood may be one of anxiety or depression and may be a chemical response to the pain itself. The affective aspect of pain often responds to antidepressants and medications that relieve anxiety.

- *Cognitive*. This is meant to convey what the pain means to you as an individual. What you think about your pain and your ideas about its cause have great influence on how much the pain will interfere with your normal enjoyment of life.

- *Behavioral*. This means what you do in response to pain, that is, your *behavior*. How you act and what you actually do to deal with your pain determine how effective your coping style will be in controlling chronic pain.

Understanding chronic pain in this way has been a major advance in our efforts to treat fibromyalgia syndrome more effectively. In the medical community this approach is generally used under the heading of "cognitive behavioral therapy."

Fibromyalgia: Fighting Back is a booklet intended to teach you to use cognitive behavioral techniques in a practical way. Being positive about your disease, establishing a proper set of goals, and developing a good coping strategy which helps you adapt rather than maladapt to your chronic pain are techniques that will predictably lead to a reduction in the severity of your illness.

Living within the boundaries set for you by your fibromyalgia will lead to an increase in daily functioning more assuredly than trying to live your life as before in spite of the illness. This of course requires an understanding of the dynamics of chronic pain and how that translates into your own personal experience of this painful condition.

It is with great pleasure that I recommend this booklet, which I hope you will find educational and enlightening. Take charge and fight back against fibromyalgia. There are many battles to be won with understanding, caring and persistence.

GLENN A. MCCAIN, MD, FRCP

ACKNOWLEDGMENTS

The author wishes to thank the following people for their encouragement and advice: Line Troster, and Fiona Graham, registered physiotherapists with a special interest in fibromyalgia; Kristin Thorson, editor of the *Fibromyalgia Network* newsletter; Mary Anne Saathoff, author of the booklet *The Fibromyalgia Syndrome;* Beth Ediger, author of the booklet *Coping with Fibromyalgia;* and Robin Saunders, program coordinator for the Ontario Fibrositis Association.

* * *

This booklet is intended to provide general information about how to cope with fibromyalgia. It is not a substitute for medical advice. Diagnosis and treatment of any symptoms or related health conditions must be provided by a physician.

A PERSONAL EXPERIENCE

When I first got fibromyalgia syndrome, I felt overwhelmed and helpless. The illness changed my life, and at first it seemed that there was nothing I could do to fight back.

Years passed before my condition was correctly diagnosed — years when everything I tried seemed only to add to my pain and debilitation. Finally an accident left me unable to walk to the corner, work or have a social life. Standing, sitting or walking produced more pain than I could handle.

Fibromyalgia is an opportunist. Following the accident it seized control of my body. I spent more than a year disabled and in great pain, dreading a single trip up the stairs, dragging myself from specialist to puzzled specialist, convinced that my life as an active person was over. I was wrong.

The day it all changed was the day I was given a name for my pain: fibromyalgia syndrome, or FMS.

Gradually I began to get the right kind of advice on what to do to fight fibromyalgia. I began to fight back. I joined an association that provided me with information and support, and learned more from other members. Because I was a writer, I worked on communications, editing the newsletter, writing a manual on how to run a support group, and making a video on fibromyalgia.

As I continued to learn about FMS, my efforts to improve my life paid off. I began to feel better.

This booklet outlines the approach that I took in overcoming many of the worst symptoms of FMS. I can now walk for blocks and blocks, sit through *Gone with the Wind*, and stand in line at the supermarket, all in the same day. I have returned to part-time work. I have learned how to pace myself, reduce some of my symptoms, and accept the symptoms that persist. My life is more satisfying and more active than it has been for years.

All this didn't happen overnight. This kind of progress cannot be bought at the drugstore. It takes work. And it usually involves false starts and setbacks as well as determination.

This is not a booklet of medical explanations and research data. I am not a doctor. I am just a person who has fibromyalgia. Like you.

I made as many mistakes as possible at every stage of my progress. Perhaps you can learn from my mistakes, and avoid repeating them.

This booklet offers you the strategy I developed for overcoming the many disabling symptoms of FMS, and accepting what could not be overcome. You will have to adapt the following battle plans to your own circumstances. Fibromyalgia is a very individual illness. It affects different people in different ways.

How many people have FMS? No one really knows, but estimates range from hundreds of thousands to millions of cases in North America alone. Some of these people experience no more than a few aches and pains. Others have the kind of life-wrecking symptoms that I have learned to fight. This booklet will be most helpful to those people who must struggle with a severe case of fibromyalgia.

These pages are a letter of hope sent to each one of you — hope that you will take the steps to better health, in your own unique way.

You have the power to improve your future.

1. AFTER THE DIAGNOSIS

I'VE GOT WHAT?

The doctor has told you that you have fibromyalgia syndrome (FMS for short). At last you have a diagnosis. That is progress. You knew there was something wrong with you and, sure enough, there is! But what is it?

Like other long medical terms, *fibromyalgia* can be broken into parts that are easier to understand. "Fibro-" means fibrous tissue, such as tendons and ligaments; "-my-" means muscle; and "-algia" means pain. Hence, pain in muscles and fibrous tissues. (In fact, the pain of FMS appears to be an 'all-over' pain sensation, described officially as 'widespread.') A *syndrome* is a group of symptoms that occur together and characterize an illness.

Knowing what the name means will give you a better understanding of your illness. However, the name does not tell you everything about fibromyalgia. This syndrome appears to affect many parts of the body. Research studies have found a wide variety of abnormalities that often occur with fibromyalgia, including a sleep disorder, imbalance in some body chemicals, and digestive problems. Not all such conditions are found in every person with FMS. Some people will have many different health problems related to fibromyalgia, while others may report only the pain and, usually, extreme fatigue at times.

The most accurate method of telling fibromyalgia from other painful conditions is finding a certain number of "tender points" in specific locations. Tender points are spots on the body that are extremely painful when pressed, though they may not hurt at other times. They occur above and below the waist and on both sides of the body *only* in fibromyalgia. Therefore they can serve as a basis for diagnosis — after tests for other possible causes of your FMS symptoms.

AT LEAST IT'S REAL

You have just lived through the toughest part of having fibromyalgia — the part where *you* know you're ill, but the rest of the human race has trouble believing it. Maybe some of your friends, or even some of your family, came to the conclusion that you were a little crazy. You had pain, fatigue, and a bewildering mix of other symptoms. You may have had diarrhea, hives or a constant sore throat. In the middle of a conversation you may have completely forgotten a point you were about to make. You may have developed a talent for dropping dishes, or had trouble focusing your eyes on the TV screen. But none of these symptoms pointed to a specific disease. Anxious trips to the doctor did not produce results. In test after medical test, you were declared completely healthy.

For every symptom, there was a logical (but unsatisfactory) explanation from other people. Pain? "You must have strained something." Exhaustion? "You've been working too hard." A rash? "You must be allergic to something." Memory lapses? "Hey, we all have those!" Dropping things? "Can't you keep your mind on what you're doing?" Diarrhea? "You ate something that didn't agree with you."

You may even have been in the miserable cycle of pain → disability → depression → more pain → more disability, a cycle that can lead you down into places no one wants to visit. Yet you couldn't explain. *It just hurt!* And no one else could see your hurt.

That's one of the worst things about fibromyalgia. It's completely invisible. It doesn't show in an X-ray or a bone scan or a standard blood test. Perhaps you feared that your problem was 'all in your head.' You may have felt guilty and ashamed. Now, thank goodness, all that is over. Your pain is real. Your other symptoms are real. It is a relief to know that you are not crazy. You are not lazy. You have a real illness called fibromyalgia syndrome.

STILL A MYSTERY

Your feelings of relief do not last long. Soon other feelings and questions may crowd into your mind. Questions like: "If fibromyalgia can be diagnosed, why didn't my doctor tell me this a long time ago, and save me all that frustration?"

Most of us believe the myth that doctors and scientists have solved all the mysteries of the human body and its ills. The truth is a little less comforting. Medical science has advanced to a remarkable degree in diagnosing and treating illness, and in understanding how the human body works. But there are still many mysteries to unravel. Fibromyalgia is one of them. Fibromyalgia is an illness with no clear cause or course. If you have been frustrated, so has your doctor. Given the incredible complexity of the illness, diagnosis is not easy. Chances are you went through an exhausting series of tests, all of them failing to find your problem. You may have frustrated more than one doctor!

Well, at least you have the right diagnosis now. You expect the usual prescription and a ten-day cure, right? Wrong.

THE GOOD, THE BAD AND THE BETTER NEWS

The good news is, fibromyalgia is not going to kill you. It is not going to put you in a wheelchair. The bad news is, there is no pill that will make it go away in ten days. There is no actual 'cure' that comes in a bottle.

Your doctor may suggest a medication that can help you get restorative sleep — the kind of sleep that helps your body heal itself. (Most people with fibromyalgia don't get this kind of sleep.) The medication will take time to work. You may have been losing restorative sleep for years. It will take much more than ten days to make up for that. If your pain levels are very high, your doctor may also suggest Tylenol or Advil or coated Aspirin to reduce the pain.

You may feel that it is almost criminal to 'take pills.' But these are not just any pills; these are medicines that a qualified physician has prescribed. Everyone needs a little help sometimes. Take them, and don't waste energy feeling guilty. The medications will not be addictive, and they should not have dangerous side effects — two important factors when considering how to manage your pain over time.

At this point your physician may explain that the treatments he or she suggests are aimed at symptom control, not at curing the condition. This sounds a little alarming.

You are going to feel better than you feel now. But more than a ten-day prescription is needed. This is going to take time. And it is going to take work!

Now here is the well-disguised better news. You can make a difference in the way you feel. You can break the vicious downward cycle (with your doctor's help).

But not just by taking pills.

The first step in fighting back is accepting that you have FMS. You have an illness that will not go away tomorrow. Acceptance does not mean defeat. Acceptance means looking your situation straight in the eye.

2. TAKING CHARGE

In the past, following your doctor's orders has produced quick results. With fibromyalgia, things are more complicated. A specialist probably won't want to see you more than once every six months. Your physician may know about fibromyalgia, but may not have the time to guide you through the steps to better health. You need to take more initiative now. You need to start helping yourself.

How?

KNOW YOUR ENEMY

Information — that's what you need first. What is this strange illness that has moved into your life?

You can get information on fibromyalgia from branches of organizations that deal with arthritis, chronic pain or chronic fatigue. Often public libraries, or the libraries of medical centres, will have literature that describes the illness and what is being done about it. Several associations of people with fibromyalgia run support groups and put out regular newsletters to keep everyone up to date.

Make contact. Join an association. Get some literature.

It will be comforting to read that certain symptoms which have puzzled you are just 'part of the package.' And you will learn that many people with severe fibromyalgia lead active, satisfying lives. They are living proof that you don't have to lie in bed for the rest of your life. Each person's story is unique. Some people with fibromyalgia go through stages when they are relatively free of symptoms. Others are able to improve their quality of life despite their symptoms. They learn how to reduce the pain, improve their sleep, and be active once again. They learn to enjoy life again. They actually have fun!

Things change. It's up to you to make them change for the better. You have already started on that road by beginning your education.

What's next?

A GOOD LISTENER

Second order of business — talk it out. You have all kinds of feelings mixed up inside. You may want to talk about your feelings and try to sort things out. You need someone to listen to you.

This can be a friend (though it's better to protect your friendships by not burdening them too much; each of them is going to be of enormous value in the months to come). Listeners can be people who also have fibromyalgia. Some associations have a buddy system in which people help each other. Others have 'hot lines' set up to help you when you are in a crisis, like a panic attack, or when a problem seems too big to handle. You will be amazed at how a sympathetic listener can help you cut a problem down to manageable size.

Even better, find a counsellor — a person trained to listen and to understand your feelings. A counsellor can be a social worker, a therapist, a psychiatrist or a psychologist. Your minister, priest or rabbi may also offer counselling.

Let yourself grieve. You have lost something precious — your good health. Ill health has walked in on you when you weren't prepared. That is not nice. It is not fair, and you are not expected to like it. It's okay to cry; it might even be necessary.

Maybe you are depressed. Depression can be caused by a chemical imbalance in your body, or it can be an understandable response to your situation. Don't let it become your constant companion. Talking about depression is a good start in fighting it. If you can't shake it, maybe your doctor will refer you for professional help.

WHY ME?

You may feel angry. It seems as if the life you once enjoyed is over. Everything has changed, and no one can tell you whether you will be able to change it back.

Indignantly you think of all your friends and acquaintances who have worked as hard, dealt with as much stress, and been in as many accidents as you have. *They* didn't get fibromyalgia. Why should you?

This is a question that can't be answered right now. Ultimately the answer doesn't matter. You've got fibromyalgia. The way you cope with it is what matters.

Perhaps you have had fibromyalgia for a long time, and it is hard to believe that you can ever feel better. You may feel hopeless as well as angry. If you feel hopeless, helpless and angry all at the same time, you are a normal human being.

TALKING TO YOUR DOCTOR

Now you need to learn to talk to your doctor clearly. You know your body better than anyone else. And only you can do things for yourself every day. You have to become a partner in your health care, helping to guide your treatment.

Make notes. Write down the things that work for you. Be specific. Choose the top three items you want to discuss the next time you see your doctor. If you provide too much information, your valuable insights may be hidden in a mass of detail. Mention the most important point first — an injury that has come back to haunt you? A strategy your doctor suggested that isn't working for you?

If your doctor can't take the time to talk with you at length, explain that you are having trouble telling him or her things that are important to you. Most doctors will hear, and stop, and listen. If you and your doctor cannot talk about your medical problems, think about getting a new doctor. Maybe your style and your doctor's style don't match.

Or your doctor might be knowledgeable about other illnesses, but less than fully informed about fibromyalgia. 'Fully informed' doctors will know the symptoms of FMS, medical treatments and self-management techniques (more on these later), and they will have access to medical updates. Not every doctor can be an expert on every illness. There are just too many! That's why you may be sent to a specialist for diagnosis or initial treatment.

However you accomplish it, find a doctor who has the expertise and the time to support you in your fight with fibromyalgia. You need a doctor on your team. Your doctor should be the one who has the whole picture of everything you are doing to cope with fibromyalgia — a sort of coach who coordinates your treatment.

GAINING PERSPECTIVE

Now that you have become a partner in your health care, you must understand what you can do and what your doctor can do about FMS.

Suppose we draw a rectangle to represent fibromyalgia. The smaller part of the rectangle represents what your doctor can do for you — for example, with a medication that helps you sleep better. The other, larger part of the rectangle represents what you can do for yourself. What this means is — you can do a lot to fight FMS. You can make an enormous difference in the way you feel.

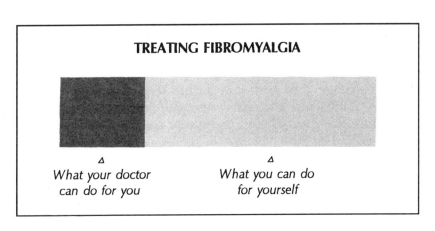

3. A MANY-SIDED APPROACH

The best results in fighting fibromyalgia come from a many-sided approach — attacking the problem from more than one angle. Pills alone won't do it. You need to know ways of coping with poor sleep, stress and perhaps many other discomforts besides pain and fatigue. FMS is a complex illness, and it affects different people different ways. Reaction to treatment tends to be individual, too. So you may find that what helps someone else is not quite right for you.

The main advice you will hear is: "You must exercise." This does not mean you should jump out of bed and run in a marathon or start weightlifting. You will have to start gradually and make sure a recommended exercise program will work for you personally.

WHY EXERCISE?

Getting as fit as you can is the best way to help your body fight this particular illness. That's why exercise will be such a big part of your treatment program.

Pain has probably made you stop exercising. Or maybe an injury or a virus stopped you in your tracks. Your muscles have become 'deconditioned' — seriously out of shape. Any form of exercise seems impossible now, and probably painful. Is it worth trying? Yes. Here's why: weakened muscles can hurt more than strong ones. Gaining muscle strength can reduce your pain, improve your overall health, and give you greater mobility. Getting stronger can help you do the things you want to do, perhaps things you thought you would never do again. Increased muscle strength and endurance can only come through exercise.

But your muscles are weak now, and they hurt. You may have tried exercise already, and gotten only more pain for your trouble. Then you had to rest to get rid of the pain. And you ended up weaker than ever!

Maybe you went too quickly. Maybe your determination took over, and you went too far. Maybe no one told you how to sneak up on your painful muscles, tendons and ligaments.

Tissues that have fibromyalgia need to be nudged gently, smoothly, gradually and systematically toward strength. Strengthening sore muscles is possible. It takes time, persistence and the correct nudging technique. Yet it can be done!

Now the only thing between you and a better-conditioned body is fear. Fear of the increased pain that exercise may bring.

LIVING WITH LESS PAIN

Relief — that's what you need! Not more pain. Perhaps even a small increase in pain from exercise is unthinkable at the moment. Yet resting can bring on more pain, too! And without the benefits of added strength and mobility.

You need a pain control strategy — some ways to decrease your discomfort *without* stopping your exercise plan.

While you are exercising, you need to listen to your body. Weak muscles get tense more easily than strong muscles. Muscle tension can lead to more pain. You need to relax all of your muscles (except the ones you are using) during exercise. Try the following suggestions.

Are you holding your breath during your exercise? That can lead to muscle tension by itself! Breathe deeply and slowly, from the abdomen. To start, try one big sigh.

Areas that need to be consciously relaxed include your shoulders, your jaw, and your facial muscles. (That grit-your-teeth grimace of determination is guaranteed to increase your pain.)

You should maintain good body posture during exercise. Unnatural weight distributions can put too much strain on sore muscles and tendons.

Use specific stretches or other exercises for the areas that hurt the most. A stretch should be smooth and gradual, held for about ten seconds, usually repeated three times. Never bounce when you stretch. Stretching muscles that have been tight for years calls for special care and patience. Check back with your doctor if even gentle stretching produces outrageous pain.

If you need more help, try applying a cold pack or a hot water bottle to the worst spots. This can work wonders.

Cold and hot packs can be bought at any back care shop. Try a bag of frozen corn if you can't afford a cold pack. A cold pack is better because it remains soft, so it can mould to your body shape straight from the freezer. But remember, never put ice or a cold pack or a *hot* water bottle directly on your skin because all of them can burn the skin. A dish towel makes a good protective layer. Use these aids for no more than ten minutes at a time (for the cold pack) or twenty minutes (for the hot pack). Longer use may cause an increase in pain.

If you hurt all over, try plunging yourself into a hot shower or a bath (with Epsom salts added) for twenty minutes. Even better, find a whirlpool bath and jet every muscle after you exercise. Use the jets sparingly at first, until you know whether your body can tolerate them. A whirlpool helps move waste products out of the muscles (along with the pain) and move fresh blood in.

Stretches or other exercises done after a hot bath or shower when the muscles are warm may bring on less discomfort than exercises done cold.

If your back, buttocks and legs are problem areas, try changing your position every twenty minutes. Get up, walk around the dining room table (or the desk, if you are at work) and then sit back down. If you can climb some stairs or march along a hallway, all the better.

Lying down for half an hour in the middle of the day can make a big difference to what you are able to accomplish in the afternoon.

Which of these strategies work best for you? Do these more often.

The fewer pills you take, the less chance there is of side-effects. While non-prescription pain relievers can be safe and useful, don't take any pills without checking with your doctor first. The main thing is to use many strategies to reduce your pain instead of relying on pills alone.

HURT WITHOUT HARM

Pain is usually regarded as a warning mechanism. We have learned to believe that pain means damage is being done. This is not always true with fibromyalgia. Your muscles may *hurt* but you may not be doing any actual *harm* to yourself. Hurt does not always mean harm. Only experience can teach you when to push past the pain and when to back off from the activity causing the pain.

What do I mean by hurt without harm?

The increased pain caused by a gradual exercise program does not necessarily point to a new injury.

Pain still sends important signals. But you have to learn a different way to read the signals. A very painful reaction to exercise that lasts for 24 hours is a 'code orange' — use caution;

you have pushed yourself too far. Reduce activity; rest the system. Unbearable pain that lasts longer than a day is 'code red' — back off, you have gone way over the line. Check with your doctor if severe pain lingers. You will be able to tell how far to go, after a while. A slight but bearable increase in pain that signals 'code green' means you are on the right track. Listening to the fear will tell you nothing. Listening to your body will tell you everything. You have to take the first step.

How?

A gentle but determined, gradual increase in physical activity, done faithfully every day, will put you on the road to strength and mobility. The rewards will outweigh the small increase in pain and, as you go, activities will become easier and more pain-free.

Your doctor or your registered physiotherapist can help you design a gradual exercise plan. One that gets you going, without bringing on a monstrous increase in pain, and without risk of injury. *Always* clear an exercise plan with your doctor before trying it. A five-minute consultation with your doctor can save weeks of discomfort. Then begin.

Inch by inch. Or house by house, as my doctor suggested.

"I can't walk to the corner," I said.

"Can you walk as far as the next house?" she asked.

"I suppose so," I said, getting suspicious.

"Then start with that. But do it every day. And then add another house. Count houses."

Naturally, I doubted this would work. But now I can measure my daily distance in blocks.

PAIN AND THE BRAIN

The way you think about your pain will have an enormous effect on the way you experience it.

The words you use matter. If you think, "I'm feeling stiff today," you minimize the message of pain. If you think, "I'm in terrible pain," you send a message through your body that will help the pain take over. A person who has 'discomfort' can live with the feeling. A person 'in pain' has few options.

Focusing your attention on the pain will not make it go away. The opposite might help, though.

Distract your mind from your discomfort whenever you can. Listen to your favourite music; read your favourite book again; watch a funny movie. (Laughter actually releases your body's natural pain-killers into your system.)

FATIGUE AND FMS

Some people who have fibromyalgia experience extreme fatigue — fatigue that cannot be ignored. It is more than feeling tired after a hard day at work. This kind of fatigue can disrupt a person's life completely. It is as serious as pain, and it can be as tough to handle.

Friends, colleagues and family may find it hard to sympathize. They might call you lazy or suggest: "*No one* needs that much rest," or "If you tried a little harder, you could do more." Such remarks are no comfort to you if you have profound fatigue. Try explaining that it is like having the worst flu in the world. Or like needing rest after working 18 hours a day for a week.

The extreme fatigue is likely to come and go, depending on how well you sleep and how you balance your activities. If it settles in for months, you may have the chronic fatigue syndrome. This has many of the same symptoms as the fibromyalgia syndrome. However, treatment for the two illnesses is likely to be different. For instance, people with chronic fatigue syndrome can rarely manage an ambitious exercise program.

Some people with FMS find that exercise begins to reduce their fatigue, especially if they can do aerobic exercise regularly. Exercise can actually give you energy!

Others find that frequent rest periods during the day keep the fatigue at bay and allow them to accomplish more than if they try to 'bull through.'

SLEEPING BETTER

You can also reduce your fatigue by getting better sleep at night. If you wake up in the morning feeling exhausted, you may not be sleeping deeply enough for your body to get 'recharged.'

Follow your doctor's advice in treating this problem. Then do everything you can to help yourself.

Improve your 'sleep hygiene.' Develop a routine that you follow every night. Read, snack and get ready for bed the same way. Go to bed at the same time, and get up at the same time every day. Avoid a daytime nap if you can because it may interfere with your sleep at night, but do try to rest during the day.

Use relaxation techniques to help you fall asleep, and be sure that you are comfortable in a good bed, with appropriate pillows. Try drinking a glass of warm milk at bedtime, and perhaps taking a hot bath to ease the pain.

Block out distracting sounds like traffic noise or family talk by using 'white noise' from a fan, or by playing a tape of surf or rain. Stay up as late as you can.

As you become more physically active, you will find you are sleeping better — another benefit of exercise!

4. GOING INTO ACTION

All the experts agree that you must exercise. *The way* you exercise can either help improve your life or bring you unwelcome misery.

ABOUT EXERCISE

Do your exercising when you are not too tired. Leave it to the end of the day, and you might well end up leaving it until the next day, and so on. A little determination goes a long way here. You need to exercise *every day*. Consider exercise a daily routine, like brushing your teeth.

But be realistic. If you aim for hours of exercise each day, you won't be able to maintain it, day after day. (And your body will almost certainly react with a long and loud 'code red'!) Start with five minutes. Wait 24 hours to see if your body is going to give you feedback. Fibromyalgia reactions often come the next day. A small, manageable increase in pain? Do the five minutes every day for a week. Then try for seven minutes, or a brisker pace. Or the same routine twice a day, then three times. . . .

A few minutes of exercise every two to three hours is much more effective than two hours once a week.

Stretching and Strengthening

If you have had a physical injury, get referred to a physiotherapist. Try to find a therapist who has already worked with people who have fibromyalgia. If he or she has not, bring along some of that literature you got. Explain clearly how long your activities have been limited and why. Exercises can be devised that work around your problem area. A combination of stretching and strengthening works best for most people with fibromyalgia.

If you have no specific physical injury, but just fibromyalgia, you must still approach exercise cautiously. Stretching is usually the first step to take before attempting other forms of exercise. A doctor or a physiotherapist can show you the right way to gradually stretch stiff and tight muscles. (Too aggressive a stretch can have the opposite effect, resulting in more stiffness.)

People with fibromyalgia should pay particular attention to the back and the neck. Your exercise expert can tell you how to strengthen the muscles that support these areas — for example, the abdominal muscles. Start with the easiest exercises and work up to the hardest. Go slowly. Give yourself time. Your muscles are sensitive.

It's important to have informed advice. How far you take it depends on your unique symptoms. Only you can tell what your body can handle.

Make a Splash at the Local Pool

Walking in the water is an ideal form of exercise. The water reduces strain on joints, while stimulating circulation. Cold water can do more harm than good, though. Find a warm pool (84ºF minimum), and start with a short, gentle dip. Walk forwards; walk backwards (always remembering to look behind you for obstacles); walk sideways. Move your arms in all directions while standing in the water up to your chin. Start with five minutes. You survived? Next time, try seven minutes.

Are there aqua-fit programs in your area? Check them out with your local fibromyalgia association or your town's recreation department. Make sure the water isn't too cold, and beware of programs geared to people who don't have FMS. Lobby for a geared-down program. Persons with arthritis or multiple sclerosis can help make up your 'gentle exercise' class. Or go it alone during 'adult swim' times. Trying to achieve gentle pool exercise while surrounded by active children is not advised.

Water exercise at least three times a week, spaced out nicely, makes for a good program. Your aim — as much as you can handle; ultimately, at least a half hour at a time, if your body can take it.

Stepping Out

Walking comes second as a great form of exercise. Running shoes with comfortable support for your arches and shock-absorbing soles will help you start walking. (Without them you may put unhealthy stress on foot or knee joints.)

Start gently, as always. Gradually work up to brisk walking of at least twenty minutes. In the winter wear clothing that will keep your muscles warm.

Aerobic Exercise

In aerobics, the idea is to increase your heart rate to a prescribed level for a certain period of time. Your doctor will advise you of the correct aerobic heart rate for your age and condition. If you can work up to 20-30 minutes of aerobics three times a week, that's great. However, some people with fibromyalgia have personal limits beyond which they cannot go. Try to get huffing and puffing for 10 minutes at least, perhaps in two sessions during a day instead of a longer session once. You will still benefit!

Move ahead at your own speed. Work up to aerobic levels gradually, but as soon as you can. This will stimulate chemical changes in your body, and can dramatically improve the way you feel all over.

Videotapes on low-impact aerobics are good to try. You can usually borrow a few from your local library, and so find out what suits you before you buy one.

Of course, you can dance around the living room to your own selection of music, or even march to a band. It's not a good idea to join a regular aerobics class unless you are in great condition and can follow the leader without difficulty.

Other Options

T'ai Chi is a stylized form of exercise developed in China. It looks easy, but it is really quite challenging. Begun gently, it could be a terrific exercise for you.

Yoga exercises are probably the most effective for stretching and keeping you flexible. However, you may have to modify the regular yoga routines to suit your ability, and work up slowly from a few minutes a day.

Manipulating chunks of Plasticine every night (as you listen to music or watch television) will do wonders for your hands. Squeezing a foam ball can also help. Massaging one hand with the other helps both hands. (More on massage later.)

Bicycling can be very beneficial, and enjoyable as well. As always, start with small doses, and increase your time gradually. Stationary bicycles should be used with zero pressure at first.

Never Give In, Never Give Up

Weekly totals of all exercise should reach three hours or more (no matter what the limit on your continuous exercise time).

You are in training, like an Olympic athlete. But the reward you're after is not just a medal, it is better health. Now *that's* something worth fighting for! So you have to be tough with yourself sometimes. But not too tough. Sound tricky?

LISTEN TO YOUR BODY!

No one else can hear what your body is saying. You alone can tell when you've pushed yourself too far — to a 'code red'. With exercise you will feel an increase in discomfort. Remember, a small increase is okay, a huge increase is not!

There is a time to fight the pain and fatigue, and a time to rest. Fibromyalgia affects each person differently. You will have to find the kind and amount of exercise that is right for you.

Usually this requires trial and error. Try to make your errors small ones.
As you progress, your exercises will become easier. They will be replaced by more challenging exercises. If you don't continue to fight FMS, you will lose ground.
The bottom line is — you should never stop exercising. The human body was designed to move and bear weight on the planet Earth. The health of muscles, tendons, cartilage and bones depend on weight-bearing and movement. Maybe your body needs a day off once in a while. But too much 'time out' will increase pain and introduce troublesome imbalances in your system.
Your body will thank you for using it!
You don't have to hurry. You just have to keep on trying. Be consistent and persistent.
Is exercise the last word? By no means. There are other simple, practical ways to help yourself.

GETTING COMFORTABLE

Strive to be as comfortable as possible in every part of your daily routine. In this way you can avoid many muscle strains and pains.

Taking A Stand

Bad posture can be a real pain. It can apply too much pressure or even a shearing force to certain parts of the body. How do you know if you have bad posture? Take this short test. Are your shoulders rounded or pushed forward? Is your chin poking up? Does your abdomen get in the way when you try to see your toes? Are your knees locked when you stand? If you answered yes to any of the above questions, you've got it — posture that can add to your pain!
Re-aligning your body (according to its original design) will ease the pain from the strained ligaments and over-worked muscles which are struggling against gravity to hold you up! Your physiotherapist or doctor will show you how to "take a good stand." Practise it until your body can remember it without an instruction manual.

Sitting Down

What is the best chair in your home or work area to sit in comfortably? A good chair is designed to provide support for your spine and your thighs so that your supporting muscles can relax.

Choose a firm seat. You may need to get an orthopedic back-rest — it can make an enormous difference. Stores that cater to people with bad backs will carry more than one design. The Obus Forme is popular, but one person's ideal back-rest can be another person's 'pain in the back.' Try them out before investing in one. If you know a friend with a back-rest, and can get visiting rights, sit and test it for at least an hour.

Some ergonomic chairs already have good back support built in. Arm rests at the correct height should support your forearms so that you can relax your shoulders. If you haven't got an armchair, put a fat pillow on your lap as an arm-rest.

Now you've got the chair and back-rest combination. But it won't do any good if you sit on the edge and slouch. Sit well back, with your buttocks against the back-rest and your back leaning against the support you have carefully chosen. Feel the difference?

The Best Beds

Before you had fibromyalgia, a good mattress was a luxury. Now it is a necessity. Deep restful sleep will give you the energy to fight fibromyalgia. Too hard or too soft a mattress will make restorative sleep impossible.

What sort of a bed do you need?

Some people swear by water-beds; some hate them. Don't consider buying one of these without a full night's trial. If none of your friends has one, find a hotel that does. The bed will cost a lot more than a night's hotel charge.

Foam mattresses are less expensive than standard mattresses. A foam mattress can be custom designed to your needs (usually with a firm core and a softer surface layer). Or try an air mattress — you can adjust the hardness of the mattress until it feels perfect.

'Egg carton' foam, or a thick wool pad like a sheep skin on top of your present mattress might be enough to do the trick. You need good support for your back, but also a surface that gives a little.

The mattress alone probably won't be enough to achieve real comfort. It might help to sleep with a pillow under your knees (when lying on your back), or between your knees (when lying on your side). This reduces the strain on your back.

You should try a cervical support pillow. This is a fancy name for a foam pillow with a ridge that supports your neck. It will keep your spine properly aligned while you are lying down. The result could be avoidance of much potential neck and back pain. Any back relief store carries a variety of these neck-support pillows, and some drugstores and department stores stock them as well. If you can, try a friend's before you buy one. Then give yourself time to get used to the pillow you choose — it will feel peculiar at first.

A CHEERING SECTION

Everyone needs the other kind of support — friendly encouragement. Go to the meetings of your local fibromyalgia association. People there will know how you feel, and encourage you. They will share information on health professionals who understand FMS, and on treatments that have worked for them. Information always helps.

If your loved ones don't understand what's happening to you, ask your doctor to speak to them. Bring them with you to your next appointment. Supply them with literature. Take them to a support group meeting.

Try to get your family into your cheering section. If you can't, work on trying to cope with the anger and disappointment you may feel.

If there is no support group in your area, consider starting one. If you can't find any other people with FMS in your area, you could still write to someone. Ask the nearest group or organization to find you a pen-pal. It's great to communicate with someone who *really* knows how you feel.

MASSAGE

A good massage by a registered massage therapist can take the kinks out of stiff muscles, relax you, and increase circulation. The massage helps push waste products (one cause of pain) out of the muscles, and bring in freshly oxygenated blood.

Unfortunately, massages cost money, and their effects don't last long.

If you can't afford more than an occasional massage, you can still use the technique to help yourself, at any time of the day or night. Many massage schools offer short programs to teach self-massage or basic massage between friends or husband and wife. For example, it is easy to massage one hand with the other, and this can sometimes bring relief. More challenging but still possible is self-massage for an arm, a thigh or a calf muscle. The very act of massaging can act as physiotherapy for your hands, and help strengthen them.

Small electric massage machines can be purchased from back care stores, and many large drugstores and department stores carry them. As with professional massage, many people with fibromyalgia say they bring great relief, while others feel they increase the pain. They are certainly worth a try.

REDUCING STRESS

Reducing stress can help you control your symptoms.

No-one can avoid stress. Sad events like the death of a friend mean stress. Even happy events like going to a party create a certain amount of stress. And pain of course generates a lot of stress all by itself.

As long as we're alive we are going to experience stress. As long as you have fibromyalgia you will have to learn to manage stress in a way that minimizes its impact on your symptoms.

Again, what you think and how you think can increase or decrease your response to stress. You can learn a new way of thinking about stress.

If there is a stress management course in your area, and you can take it, do so. Can't go to a course? Borrow a book from the library on the subject. There are many good ones.

Even before the class begins or you read the book, try this simple technique to reduce the effects of stress. Change your shallow, rapid breathing (a sure sign of stress) to deep, slower breathing. Breathe from the abdomen several times, making your belt tighten and loosen with each breath. Put a slight smile on your face and say to yourself, "Mind amused; body relaxed."

Okay, it sounds silly. But this 'seven-second method' can begin to reduce the physical affects of tension.

Not good enough? Here are some more methods to try.

Finding Your Stress Factors

Certain people, situations or events will make you feel anxious, irritable or downright angry. Ask yourself, "What are the things that upset me most?" The answers will reveal some of your stress factors.

What now? Take those stressful things out of your life as much as you can. Just get rid of them! The result? Less stress!

Can't get rid of them? Talk to your counsellor, minister or telephone buddy about them. See if you can take some of the aggravation out of them. You can learn to react differently to these difficult situations. While you're working on this, try to encounter those upsetting events or people less often.

We have much more control over our lives than we think. Each of us can learn to assert that control.

The very thought that you can control a stressful situation lessens the adverse effects of stress. Stress for bosses, for example, is often less damaging than for the workers they supervise. This is because bosses have some control of circumstances at work, while those working for them are often powerless to do anything about a bad situation.

PLANNING YOUR DAILY LIFE

By now you are beginning to find out how many activities you can handle in one day. Trying to do too much will certainly bring on more fatigue and additional pain. Avoid these problems by planning your daily life. Try to arrange your schedule within the limits of your energy. Can you manage only two things on a particular day? Put off the third. Don't put yourself in an overload situation. Save your energy for the things that really need to be done or the activities you like best.

Do you find it difficult to keep track of what you are supposed to do? Buy a notebook or a large calendar and write down the times and dates of your activities. If you have a lot of demands on your time, try using an appointment diary for reminders to yourself.

Schedule rest time into each day. You know how much you need. Adjust your schedule until you can get it. If you can't rest one day, anticipate fatigue the following day and cancel as much on that day as you can.

If profound fatigue is a frequent problem, you need to build flexibility into your schedule. Tell friends or family that you will try to make it to an outing, but warn them that you may not be able to. It will depend on how you feel that day. Some people find that their fatigue is so unpredictable that they must often cancel plans. Even if you feel well when you are on the way to an event, fatigue or pain may waylay you later. Think ahead. Is there a couch or bed available for rest where you are going? Will the host or hostess be horrified if you need to lie down? Will you have a chance to move around if necessary? Check out the situation and make a decision that you can live with. The formal dinner-dance or banquet might not be possible for you. The casual get-together at your mother's house might be fine. Planning ahead will avoid an embarrassing moment, or increased discomfort.

Don't forget to include fun times in your plans. Just knowing a pleasant event is coming can create cheerful anticipation for weeks. On the other hand, you may have to miss some activities that you love. That is unfortunate, but you have to consider whether a particular activity is worth the price you are going to pay for it. Maybe it is! Do it, then, but schedule in a day of rest after it.

As you get stronger you will probably be able to re-introduce more activities into your schedule. At first, take it slowly, don't over-commit yourself. And allow for delays by leaving a little early for appointments. Rushing is a guaranteed stressor.

MANAGE YOUR MEMORY

Many people who have fibromyalgia have trouble remembering or concentrating. Sometimes they lose track of a conversation, or they feel disoriented in familiar places. They get directions wrong. They forget appointments. They 'misplace' the names of persons they know perfectly well, or switch letters or words around by mistake. Their short-term memory is often affected. They may forget the name of a person they just met, for example, but not something like the name of their home town, which is established in long-term memory.

These are small things, taken one at a time; quite terrifying if they are all happening to you at once.

For some, this is almost as bad as the fatigue, the pain, the irritable bowel or the clumsiness that can be part of fibromyalgia. For some, there is nothing more frightening than feeling you are 'losing your mind.'

You are not losing your mind. (By all means discuss this fear with your doctor, though.) The panic you feel is completely normal. Anyone in the same circumstances would feel the same. But don't give in to the panic.

You *can* do something about your memory. The following are a few suggestions.

o Manage your fatigue better. Your mind does not operate in isolation from your body — both need energy to do work. When you are well rested you will likely find it easier to concentrate. Just one night of disturbed sleep can reduce anyone's mental performance. You have probably had disturbed sleep for many nights.

o Talk to your doctor about your fatigue and sleep patterns. You may be taking a medication that produces fatigue, mind fog or loss of short-term memory. Changing the time when you take it can minimize these problems.

o Concentrate on only one thing at a time. This sounds absurdly simple, but it isn't. Don't think about other things while balancing your cheque book, for example. If other thoughts interrupt while you are trying to concentrate, and you don't want to forget them, *stop*. Write them down; then get back to the task at hand.

o Get rid of distractions. Distractions can destroy your ability to concentrate. Turn off the radio when you want to read or have a conversation. Clean up the clutter where you live or work; it is a visual distraction. If you can't decide what to do with the clutter, scrunch it into one neat pile, or a file marked 'To sort.' Put bills in a separate pile, with their due dates clearly visible.

o Do your most demanding mental work at the time of day when you are most alert. This time will vary from person to person.

o Schedule rest for your mind into your day. You need it just as much as physical rest. Silence can be wonderfully restorative in our over-stimulated society.

o Handle pain in the best way you and your doctor have devised. Simply being in pain can drain you of the energy you need to think clearly. This includes emotional pain. Feeling depressed or worrying about your future can affect your ability to think.

o Talk about your worries. Learning to let go of them may make more 'mental space' available. You might try writing your worries down in a special diary. Then your concerns are recorded; you don't need to keep them on a repeating tape in your mind. Exploring ways to solve some of your problems on paper can help you take the appropriate action.

o Use the kitchen timer or a beeper on an inexpensive watch to remind you of critical things in your day.

o Add texture to the things you want to remember. For example, remember a name by learning about the person's hobbies or job, and see if you have something in common. Repeat the name often aloud and to yourself. Link the sound of the name with an object in your mind. Write it down. This is called deeper processing. By adding information associated with the name, you make the name easier to recall. Memory aids like rhymes or acronyms can also help.

Exercise your mind on as regular a schedule as you exercise your body. You may need to use graduated mental exercises, just as you used graduated physical exercises. Your ability to concentrate should increase as you practise. Stimulation alone is useful.

Each person's problems and solutions are unique. If you are still having a lot of trouble with your memory after following the above suggestions, tell your doctor. Other methods of improving your memory do exist. Ask for 'cognitive restructuring' or 'cognitive stimulation' exercises if you need more help. Or play more games. Many board games offer excellent mental exercise.

Slow down. Give yourself time. Pressure can only interfere with recall. A little patience and a sense of humor can help a lot. Joke about your memory lapses, and people will laugh with you. Everyone forgets things.

LEARNING TO LET GO

You have gotten rid of as many stressful situations as you can. Now you have to learn to live with the rest. Your response to each stressor, especially your response to pain, will make a difference. You need to learn to relax. And the 'seven-second relaxation' is not enough.

Relaxation

Your stress management course or book should talk about relaxation methods. Just reading about them will not change your life. You have to practise. Save half an hour every day for relaxation. Buy a relaxation tape and listen to it daily. Or practise the method taught in your course every day, until you can use your relaxation method anywhere, any time you need it.

You may have to try several methods of relaxation before you find the one that 'fits' you. There are many ways to relax. Perhaps lying on the couch, listening to soothing music, works for you. Because you are not as physically active as you used to be, and because you have pain, relaxation may not be easy. But it is achievable.

And don't let your time for relaxation get cut out of your day. It is vital to your recovery.

Don't hurry, don't worry. Stop fearing the future and mourning the past for just half an hour. (Stop it all the time, if you can!) You can only live in the present, and do the best you can today.

In spite of your best efforts, though, you may find that tension accumulates. We all have muscle groups that tend to 'carry' our tension. Relaxing your muscles may help to reduce your pain. Stop muscle tension before it stops you.

Self-Biofeedback

Self-biofeedback is a simple technique of listening to the feedback or the messages from your body. You can often halt escalating pain by doing a *seven-point check* at intervals through the day.

1. Check your shoulders. Have they started to creep up toward your ears? Gently but firmly pull them down and stretch them back, pulling your shoulder blades together, shrugging them, moving them in circles until they have relaxed.

2. Check your jaw. Is it clenched? Part your teeth without parting your lips, rest your tongue on the roof of your mouth and relax your jaw muscles.

3. Check your neck. Is it held rigidly in one position? Take a moment to stretch your neck muscles in all directions (easy, gradual stretches).

4. Check your back. Is your chair providing adequate support? Are you leaning back in the chair, using that support, or are you hunched forward? Correct your posture. It may help to stand up and walk a few steps.

5. Check your legs. Are they relaxed and comfortable, or have you tensed them in one position? A foot support, such as a telephone book, can allow you to let your leg muscles go. A real foot-rest at the right angle and height is not too costly. Buy it at your local back-care store and move it from chair to chair.

6. Check your forehead. Are you frowning? Try to rid your face of all expression, then replace the frown with a slight smile. Feel that your tongue and your ears are loose.

7. Straighten your arms. Flex your fingers into fists and out again several times. Rotate your wrists. Shake your hands as if flicking water off them. This is especially useful if you have been writing or typing.

Breathe deeply during the above checks, and several times at the end of the process. Use the seven-second relaxation technique, ending with a big sigh.

Soon you will detect muscle tension before it builds up, and be able to release it quickly. You will identify your own personal tension patterns, and adapt the check list to your unique needs.

You are regaining control over your body. You are making fantastic progress.

5. ASSESSING YOUR LIFE

Whatever your type of work, you may have to take some time off because of the effects of fibromyalgia.

If you work at being a homemaker and have young children, time off will not come easily. See if a relative or friend can take over for a while each day, so you can schedule rest and exercise. If you don't take care of yourself now, pain and fatigue may force you to stop doing everything later. You are as important as any other member of your family. And you are much more important than a clean house.

If you are studying at school, memory lapses and fatigue will be particularly distressing. See whether you can reduce the number of classes you take. Part-time studies might be possible. Don't neglect your physical self when pushing to finish an assignment on time. Perhaps your doctor would be willing to explain your situation to the teachers, instructors or professors.

If FMS has struck you during your retirement years, you may be unable to fulfill your retirement dreams. Plans might have to be changed. You and your companion will have to work out just what is possible for you. Since you likely have the time to manage your illness, you should be able to improve your health over a period of months. Soon you will be able to take on more activities.

If you have been working outside the home and can no longer hold down a paying job, the uncertainty and sudden loss of employment can be devastating. Many people identify with their jobs. You thought of yourself as a carpenter, steelworker, bus driver, teacher, manager, or nurse. Your job had probably become familiar and comfortable. It gave you an identity, the friendship of fellow workers, a feeling of self-worth and a sense of purpose. Society judged you by the job you had and what you earned.

YOUR SELF-ESTEEM

Loss of your main occupation can be a big blow to your self-esteem. You feel a loss of control over your life, and you don't know if you will ever be better. You may have feelings of uselessness, isolation, boredom, guilt, depression. This deadly combination can sap your strength, just when you need it most. No one told you fibromyalgia would be like this!

Turn it around. Imagine that your best friend is facing your situation. What would you say to him or her? Say those things now to yourself. "You are more than your work. You are more than a batch of symptoms."

Recovering a sense of self-worth won't happen overnight. Don't give up on it, though. Feeling good about yourself will help you to move from being a victim to being a victor. You may not get rid of your fibromyalgia. But you can get back your self-respect.

YOU AND YOUR JOB

Many people with fibromyalgia find they can return to their old jobs as long as the jobs are not too physically demanding. Some people have to find different jobs — for example, jobs that create less stress. Some may have to work part-time. And some will find it extremely difficult to work at any structured job with a regular schedule. It will take time to learn what you yourself can do.

Your specialist or your doctor may be able to make intelligent guesses as to how long you will need to follow a reduced schedule (both mentally and physically). But these are only guesses. It will take months of consistent effort to reach your plateau — the level of activity that you, your mind and your body can tolerate.

Perhaps you will find that you can no longer do as much for your family as you used to. Other members of your family may have to take on more tasks. It can be difficult for spouse and children to understand why you can't carry on as before, when you 'look so well.' An uncomfortable period of adjustment can be helped by family discussions.

If you cannot hold down a paying job, another problem may be about to surface. Financial worries may add to your stress, and therefore add to your fibromyalgia symptoms. Other members of the family may have to work more to compensate. Or you and your family may have to give up things that you could once afford. Inquire about other forms of income, like disability pensions and compensation payments. Do you qualify for any of these?

Questions like that can alarm the strongest person. It's very scary to admit that you might not be able to do your 'normal' work. In most places it is very difficult to get any kind of compensation for disability caused by fibromyalgia alone. But if your fibromyalgia was triggered by an accident on the road or at work, you may have a stronger legal case for compensation.

Think of your inquiries as a way of storing up ammunition that may or may not be used in the future. If finances are a big problem *now*, ask a friend to help you explore your options. Solutions exist, even when we feel they do not.

You may have to change your job, live an entirely different kind of life! This seems overwhelming right now, but there are experts who can help.

WHAT ARE YOUR OPTIONS?

Hospitals, mental health centres, or even the YM/YWCA can provide guidance. Your local library or community college can help you find a new vocation. You may have to start again to consider your options and your aptitudes. Government employment centres and some industries may offer both assessment and training programs in your area. Look into them. This will take time. Be prepared to make about ten phone calls to arrive at a single answer. Do this while lying down, or in the most comfortable chair you own! If you were injured on the job, your union or a compensation board may provide similar services, and could act as advocates to get you back to work gradually, on a modified work schedule. There may be government initiatives to employ the physically disabled in your area. Try not to panic at the word 'disabled.' Your doctor will help determine if you are indeed in this category.

As you work on your health, and you begin to feel better, volunteer work could act as a bridge leading back to paid employment. Volunteer work will bolster your self-esteem and bring you into contact with other people, reducing your isolation. Certainly it is a satisfying and worthwhile activity in its own right.

Take time to consider your choices. Don't make any major decisions in a hurry.

PARDON ME, BUT YOU'RE STEPPING ON MY DREAMS

Fibromyalgia does more than disrupt your life. It disrupts your dreams — goals that you set for yourself before all this happened. Perhaps they included a job that you intended to win through hard work and perseverance, or that trip around the world that you had been putting off until a convenient time. We all cherish secret desires that we hope to make happen in the future. But now you don't know what your future will be like.

ADJUSTING YOUR EXPECTATIONS

You need a new plan, a new point of view. You have changed. You must look at things differently.

You have been fighting an illness. Now you are feeling better. But better than what? If you focus on your life 'before fibromyalgia', you will continue to feel sad. Don't compare your present level of activities to what used to be 'normal' before you got fibromyalgia. Focus on your functioning, not on your pain. If you focus on what you *can* do now, you will start to feel better. If you need a benchmark to use as a comparison, use the point at which you were most disabled, most helpless. Without your hard work, you might still be that way today. You have improved. That is wonderful!

Assessing Your Life

You may have to change your expectations. This is a tough one. We all want to get back everything. We all want to be 'normal', or what we consider normal.

Look at it this way. Fibromyalgia used to run your life. In the diagram below, the small centre of the first circle represents the part of your life that you were controlling when you first began to fight back. The big, shaded portion shows how much of your life fibromyalgia was controlling. Little by little, you've been taking back control of your life. Now you are running much more of the show, as in the circle on the right. Even if you don't completely get rid of FMS, you have made tremendous progress.

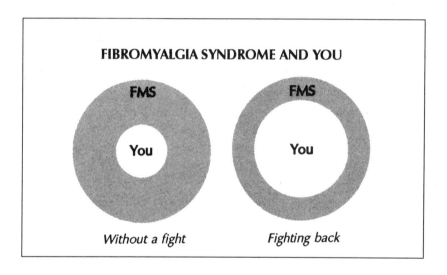

Pare down your expectations until they are realistic. Work toward your more realistic goals. Sadness and anger may surface from time to time. These feelings are real; they are natural; they are human. Pay them as much attention as they need, and then go on.

Life has changed. But it still has many good things in it. You may have to move at a slower pace from now on. But you're still moving!

When your expectations are closer to your present abilities, you will have fewer disappointments, and more fun.

6. FROM VICTIM TO VICTOR

People who passively accept FMS seldom get better. People who fight back can improve their lives. You don't have to spend the rest of your life feeling like a victim. Be a victor instead!

TAKING STOCK

Celebrate your victories! Take time to savour each step forward. The journey back to better health is not easy. You deserve a lot of credit. But there may be some things you don't feel like celebrating.

You've gone through the steps. You've given the strategy a fair chance. But now you may see that you will not regain all that you lost through FMS. For some, this is reality.

It hurts. It feels like a failure. "If only I had done this or that; if only I *hadn't* done that other thing!" These 'if only's' can be deadly. We can't rewrite our personal history.

First, stop blaming yourself. You did not invite FMS into your life. The limitations on what you can do are not your fault. Reality may be painful right now, but you haven't failed. On the contrary, you have changed what could be changed; you have moved your body toward wellness; now you recognize what cannot be changed. (At least, not now. As medical research progresses, a cure for fibromyalgia may be found. Even without a cure, new treatments should become available that will at least reduce your symptoms.)

Next, stop blaming fate or the person who triggered your FMS by running into your car. Blame takes energy. You can't spare your energy. You need it all to live.

Now you have to begin letting go of some of the things that you cannot recover. This is more painful, for some, than that first period of doubt and depression. Don't expect to heal overnight. But you now know about the tools that can help you heal — new ways of coping, new attitudes. As soon as you can, start using them.

REMEMBER TO HAVE FUN

Some of the things you used to enjoy may be difficult or even impossible for you to do now. But there must be *some* enjoyable activities you can still do. DO THEM! Don't let your difficulties divert you totally from living your life. Whether it's reading a book or listening to music — do it! And once in a while go out and do something challenging but wonderful. You may have a bad day afterwards, but the sense of freedom and satisfaction in enjoying life will be worth it.

LAUGHTER IS POWERFUL MEDICINE

Watching a funny movie, chuckling over a joke, smiling over the cartoons in the newspaper — these should be part of your prescription for health. Cut out the best cartoons and tape them up. Laughter heals. It affects the immune system and releases beneficial chemicals into the body. Even if laughter can't defeat every symptom of fibromyalgia, you should do it just because it feels good!

SOME DIET TIPS

The best diet for FMS is no diet. You should eat a variety of foods including fruits, vegetables, whole grains and proteins, so as to give your body the nutrition it needs.

If for some reason you are not able to eat certain foods, a doctor may recommend a 'one-a-day' vitamin capsule. But a varied diet should supply all the vitamins your body can absorb and use.

Many 'health foods' may be wholesome, but they are also expensive, and you probably don't need them. Beware of fad diets, supplements and 'cures' recommended by people with no medical training.

Different people react differently to different substances. If you have breast or chest wall pain, try cutting out caffeine; you may get relief and also find yourself less jumpy.

Do try to keep your weight within the recommended range for your age and height. You should be aware that some medications prescribed for you may cause you to gain or lose weight. If this is a serious problem for you, you might ask your doctor to let you try another medication in the same 'family' of drugs instead. With luck, the new medication will not have the same effect.

Some people who have FMS are very sensitive to caffeine or milk products, or perhaps to other foods or alcohol. This seems to fall in the same category of being more sensitive to all environmental factors — like smoke, noise, cold and bright light.

If you suspect you have some food sensitivities, begin keeping a diary of what you eat. Write down how you feel a few hours afterwards. Over time you may be able to link an allergic reaction or digestive irritation to specific foods and beverages. Of course you should consult your doctor about any ongoing discomfort.

THE "HOW ARE YOU?" TRAP

People are going to ask how you are. They are sincerely interested. But they don't want a detailed lecture on fibromyalgia, or the fine points of an irritable bowel. This is a sort of minefield in human relations for anyone with a chronic ailment.

You may not want to think about how you are. Ignoring certain things may be a legitimate coping technique (after you have done what you can). You want to think about other things — cheerful things, the good parts of being alive. But people are still going to ask. You need to work out a few answers that are neither outright lies (this is damaging to yourself) nor lengthy explanations.

Here are some suggestions. "A little sore today, but in general pretty good." "Not too bad. Getting better." "I haven't quite made it yet, but I'm working on it." Then there's "Pretty good" on its own, or "Better than yesterday," or "This isn't one of my best days." How about, "It's great to see you! I'm glad to be back in circulation." The thing to do is to give as honest an answer as possible, while avoiding the details that seem essential (to you), and boring (to most other people). Also, the answers you give to other people are easily detected by your own ears. Give yourself a positive message as much as possible.

Gracefully sum up your situation while deflecting further questions. If you're about to see some people after a long absence, get these answers ready in advance. Nothing can block creative thinking like an earnest inquiry after your health.

LEARNING TO SAY NO

Because you look completely 'normal,' people are going to ask you to do things that will cost your body more than you are prepared to pay. Even people close to you, who know you well, will slip up from time to time. Be tolerant! It is just incredibly hard for anyone else to understand what you are going through.

You need to learn to say no with grace. This is a real challenge. There must be no hurt feelings or sloppy emotions left after the crucial encounter.

Try some of the following:
- "I am so pleased you asked me!" (Okay, this may be a little white lie, but it's in a good cause.)
- "I would really like to help out, but I'm totally booked up that week." (You are booked up. You have some essential relaxation to attend to.)
- "This is a great thing you are doing. I wish you the best. Unfortunately I can't be a part of it this time, but I'll be more than happy to donate a couple of dollars." (Accompanied by a smile. The smile is important.)
- "Not Wednesday night! Oh, I'm sorry, I'm booked." (For an early night's sleep.) This one should be used with caution. If the event can be shifted, you may suddenly have to invent a different excuse. Perhaps the safest is the one closest to the truth.
- "I would really like to, but I'm not quite up to that much activity yet."

Whatever you say, resist all efforts to instill guilt into your normal-looking breast. You worked hard to feel better. You have a right to defend your health. You don't need to apologize to anybody. Exercise, rest and relaxation are essential parts of your life. You cannot compromise on these issues.

Defend your time at all costs, because of the price you will be paying if you don't. If you don't take care of yourself, you will soon be unable to do *anything* for *anybody*. You need that healthy 'selfishness' which means looking after your health first.

FMS AND INTIMACY

No one wants to talk about the way FMS affects sex. But everyone wants to hear about it.

Sex is an important part of intimate relationships. When people lose their self-esteem and are in constant pain, it should come as no surprise that they have a reduced interest in making love. Preoccupation with health issues is natural. Bodily changes may make a person feel shy and inadequate. And the fight for better health may leave people with fibromyalgia too tired to do anything else. A serious attack of FMS fatigue will do the same thing. So some people with FMS, even if they would like to make love, may be too exhausted to make the effort.

The sexual partner of anyone with fibromyalgia still needs and wants physical intimacy.

What can be done?

You may have to schedule a rendezvous. Plan it for the time of day when you are most energetic, and most pain-free. Rest in advance; save up some energy. Give this side of your life the attention it deserves. Once you make it a priority, you may be able to rediscover the physical intimacy that was so enjoyable in the past. If certain positions are painful, experiment. Find ways of being intimate without bringing on unbearable pain. The local branch of your arthritis society may have a useful pamphlet on this subject.

Like any physical exercise, making love may leave you with slightly increased pain. The pleasure of it and the closeness to your partner may outweigh this disadvantage.

Having a partner who is chronically ill is difficult. Some mates of people with FMS will adapt easily to the necessary lifestyle changes. Some will not.

Talk about it. Look for ways to compromise. Don't hesitate to consult your doctor. Your relationship may need help in this area.

OTHER PEOPLE HURT TOO

Helping someone else can help to heal yourself. There are lots of people with problems much worse than yours. Get involved in your local fibromyalgia association. Give a little time and energy to other people. Even with your limitations, you can do this. If you can't move around much yet, you can still use a telephone. Every association needs a telephone committee. Help out as you can. A sense of perspective and a feeling of increased self-worth will be your rewards.

And don't forget about the heartache of those who love you. Tell them how much you appreciate their support and their patience. And try to understand when they appear thoughtless. If you didn't have fibromyalgia, would you believe in it?

SURVIVING THE UPS AND DOWNS

You are going to make mistakes. No insult intended, but FMS is a subtle and devious enemy. Just when you're doing well, you may have a sudden relapse. Maybe you got too confident, and overdid some activity. There may be no reason at all that you can find for an unexpected flare-up.

Suddenly, here you are again, angry, frustrated, and in more discomfort than you can handle. Blaming yourself will only make it worse. You wanted to go that extra mile — this is natural, this is part of your positive attitude.

Don't abandon the attitude. If you need more help, go and get it! Get in touch with a counsellor or a sympathetic friend as soon as possible and talk about your feelings.

Work out a crisis plan with your physiotherapist and doctor — a combination of rest and activity that will minimize your time away from your routine. It may be that you need total rest for a day or two. It may be that certain stretches and hot baths can help you get mobile again quickly.

Keep saying to yourself, "This will pass." You won't lose all you have worked for in these setbacks. Instead, the hard work you have done will help you recover sooner.

Most important of all, forgive yourself. You are only human.

YOU CAN FIGHT FIBROMYALGIA

Reading good advice is easy; living with fibromyalgia is more difficult. This booklet has touched on the issues you will face. It has pointed out some tactics to use in your fight against fibromyalgia.

I believe they can help you to improve, no matter how FMS has affected you personally.

When you begin the fight against FMS, you join the ranks of a very special group of people — people who have had the will power to make their lives better not just for one day but for the rest of their lives.

You can be a part of this group. How do I know? Many other people very like yourself have fought back to the point where they feel better, where they have regained control of their lives. You need only enough strength to take the first step today. One day at a time; one step at a time. You have already taken the first step — you have read this booklet! Take the second step, then. Worry about the third step tomorrow.

By choosing to fight fibromyalgia you have placed yourself on the winning team. Your life, and the lives of those you love, will be the better for it.